I0486129

Small Cell Lung Cancer:

Treatment Options and Alternative Medicine

Author & Published By: Natures Blueprint Nutraceutical Research Company

Publication Date: 2015

First Edition

Table of Contents

What Can These Treatments Do?

1. Can be used safely with or without Chemotherapy with an average of chemotherapy being 100% more effective and with less side effects or use the 6 agents without chemotherapy as a standalone alternative treatment.

2. Adiposis- Increases cancer cell death/ P53 activation/cell cycle arrest

3. Inhibition of cancer cell division

4. Decreases cell growth- Shrink Tumors

5. Inhibition of cell survival- Suppress new tumors/inhibit tumor cell proliferation

6. Angiogenesis- Inhibits growth of blood vessels to tumors

7. Autophagy-when cancer cells eat themselves

8. Inhibition of metastasis- Cancer Spread

9. Anti-inflammatory

10. Inhibition of carcinogens

11. Reverse/Stop drug resistance from occurring

12. Reverse/Stop Cachexia- Wasting away of the cancer patient's body

13. Reverse/Stop the fermentation process

14. Neutralize the lactic acid (which is actually what causes the cancer cells to multiply uncontrollably) and make cancer cells nontoxic/neutralized.

15. Increase the cellular oxygen levels in body

16. Balance your body's PH levels and Alkaline the cancer cells to self-destruct

17. Survival signal deactivation- For people that smoke, nicotine sends a signal to the cancer to keep growing.

18. Increase your appetite, taste buds, energy levels and bowel movements since constipation is a side-effect of pain medication, chemotherapy and overall cancer.

Studies prove at a minimum to Double or Triple life expectancy of small cell cancer patients without Chemotherapy. Some patients do have full remission for as long as 9 years. It all depends on the age of the person, prior health issues and how well treatments are tolerated.

Introduction To Small Cell Lung Cancer

Lung cancer is considered as one of the most common types of cancer in the world. This is basically categorized in two type small lung cancer and non-small lung cancer respectively. Physician can determine the type of the lung cancer the person has which may depend according to the appearance, size and behavior. 15 percent of people suffering from lung cancer has this type and the remainder as the non-small type of this cancer.

The people who are prone in developing this type of cancer are smokers mainly heavy smokers as well as former smokers. Small cell lung cancer is basically an aggressive type of cancer that grows and can spread to the system fast. This makes this type of cancer very dangerous if not diagnosed or treated right away. Many physicians agree that a surgery to remove the cancer cell is the best way to be treated right away but in most cases it cannot be treated in this way unless caught very early on before any spread and/or depending on the location.

SMALL CELL LUNG CANCER CLASSIFICATION

Just like any type of cancer, small cell lung cancer also has its classifications. The stages of cancer can determine what type of treatment, procedures or care that the patient needs. In order to determine the small cell lung cancer stage, the doctor will perform several imaging test such as CT scan (computed tomography). MRI scan (magnetic resonance imaging), PET scan (position emission tomography), bone scan and other tests. Additionally, the doctor may perform a number of biopsies to determine if the cell is cancerous or not on a certain site. The stage of small cell lung cancer is very important as this will surely help the doctor on how to effectively determine the right treatment for a person who is diagnosed with lung cancer.

Moreover, the doctor may also need to perform several tests such as blood test, urine, stool and even electrocardiogram to determine also the overall health of his or her patient. This will also play a great role for the doctor to effectively determine the methods of treatment needed by the patient.

Patient who have this condition are classified traditionally as limited-stage disease or extensive-stage disease. On the other hand, medicine experts has recommended that this kind of cancer should be classified with the same classification just like the non-small cell lung cancer with certain classification such as stage I, stage II, stage III and stage IV. This is believed to be an ideal way to have the right assessment when it comes to the extent of this condition. This will also give the expert

Limited Stage Disease – This is a stage of the cancer wherein the cancer is just affecting one lung or it is just within the mediastinum lymph nodes or the middle area within the lungs and chest. If the patient is under this stage, it also indicates that the stage is just within the range such as stage I-III as a much detailed means to determine the system of staging the condition. Moreover, one third of individuals suffering lung cancer has limited stage disease usually when diagnosed. On the other hand, in most cases, the cancer might have already spread within the chest area but may not be determined through imaging tests. This means, the doctor may need to perform additional tests to tell if there's indeed a presence of cancer cells within the chest.

Most of the individual under this stage of lung cancer are primarily treated with the use of chemotherapy or combining radiation therapy that are directed through the chest. After several initial treatments the patients are also treated with radiation therapy that is focused on the brain. This helps to prevent brain metastases as well as to prevent the development of the cancer and t be able to effectively enhance the chance to survive. The main treatment goal for patient suffering on this stage of cancer is for them to be able to be cured from cancer.

When it comes to patient with an early stage of small cell lung cancer primarily stage 1 wherein the site of the cancer cell is just on one lung, the doctor may require a surgery to remove it and in some situation, surgery is followed by chemotherapy. On the other hand, radiation therapy may not be required anymore.

Extensive-stage disease – For patients who are diagnosed small cell lung cancer with extensive stage after the initial diagnosis, it only means one thing and that the disease has already grown to its advanced stage. This is also an indication that the cancer cells have already spread to other lung tissue or has moved to other locations of the body. The common sites wherein cancer cell may spread are bones, adrenal glands and liver. The only treatment option for patient suffering from this stage is chemotherapy. Surgery is already out of the equation as this may only boost the cancer cells to move easily to other parts of the body. At this stage of small cell lung cancer, it is a stage wherein the cancer is no longer curable. The main goal of this treatment is just to relieve the symptoms and make the patient feel a bit better, so that the patient can live longer. Additionally, patients with good response to chemotherapy are often given radiation therapy especially to brain in order to prevent the cancer to metastasize in the brain. This is also used to treat other parts of the body wherein the cancer has already spread.

CHEMOTHERAPY

One of the common and most prominent types of treatment for any type of cancer is the chemotherapy. Chemotherapy is the use of various medicines in order to destroy the cancer cells and prevent them from growing. When it comes to small cell lung cancer, it is the most preferred kind of treatment. This kind of treatment works by effectively interfere the capacity of the fast growing cells to split and reproduce. Since the normal cell of an adult individual is not growing anymore, it will not be affected by this chemotherapy but not in the case of bone marrow, wherein it is the producer of blood cells. As a result, patients undergoing chemotherapy may experience the certain side effects that are not that advantageous to overall health. The side effect of chemotherapy can be seen as the treatment progresses.

There are myriad of chemotherapy active drugs that are being used to battle the small cell clung cancer and many new drugs are also being explored to test if they are effective or not. The patients suffering from this condition may be treated with one chemotherapy drug but to increase the effectiveness, the patient are usually give two drugs for chemotherapy, With the combination of two chemo drugs, it has a strong chance or opportunity to reduce the size of the cancer cell. As a result, the patient will also have a longer life or even survival especially for the patients who were diagnosed on early stage. Chemotherapy is typically administered through an injection or through IV or intravenous. Some chemotherapy drugs are also available via oral medications as well.

In general, chemotherapy treatment is administered on a weekly period, wherein the patient will require taking the chemotherapy injection or drugs for at least 2-4 days then after 3 weeks period, the phase will start again. This is also called as cycle. This period is essential for the reason that it is an ideal way on how one will able to determine the effects of chemotherapy and it is also the best way to know if there are some changes.

Duration of treatment - When it comes to the duration of chemotherapy, the doctor will first conduct an initial chemo treatment. This will help him or her to determine how the patient is responding to this treatment primarily his or her system. There are 4-6 initial chemo treatments as recommended. On the other hand, additional chemotherapy cycles may be needed in order to increase the survival rate of the patient.

Limited-Stage Disease – Patients with limited stage small cell lung cancer are commonly treated by using chemo drugs such as etopsoside (VP-16,Vepesid) and cisplatin (Platinol). As the side effect rate of cisplatin is very strong, carboplatin (paraplatin) is used as an alternative and it is believed to be same effectiveness, which is a good alternative.

Extensive-Stage Disease – When it comes to patient with the advanced stage of small cell lung cancer, the chemotherapy drugs that are used are carboplatin, cisplatin or combination of irinotecan (Camptosar), etposide. It also shows that for Japanese patients, irinotecan are more effective for them instead of etopiside. On the other hand, Caucasian patients have demonstrated good benefits with less noted side effects.

Side Effects – Since chemotherapy medication affects the normal cell of the body, it can be resulted in wide side effects. When the patient is receiving chemotherapy, the doctor needs to monitor the patient for the side effects present.

The drop in blood count as an effect of chemotherapy drugs to bone marrow is one of the primary side effects of small cell lung cancer chemotherapy. This basically happens, one or two weeks after the patient receives his or her chemotherapy. It is important for the secondary healthcare provider or the family member of the patient to report any chills or fever, which may led the person to develop certain infection like pneumonia.

Other possible chemotherapy side effects are decreased appetite, mouth sores, diarrhea, hearing loss, pain or numbness of fingers or toes, vomiting, nausea, hair loss and fatigue. It may also include decrease in appetite, kidney failure and others.

Radiation Therapy

Radiation therapy is typically recommended in the course of chemotherapy for individuals with small, limited-stage cancer. This is commonly done through using x-rays of high energy focused on a particular body part where the disease is situated, aiming of killing cancer cells. The x-rays used are delivered through a machine which is refereed as linear accelerator. The process is done externally with brief individual treatments, usually 10-15 minutes. Patients who undergo such process will not experience any kind of pain.

Radiation delivers damaging effect which is quite cumulative. Cancer cells will not eventually die just after one treatment. Typically, a certain number of radiation therapy varying from the recommendation of a physician, will be needed before a cancer cell finally die. Usually, small doses of the treatment are administered either on a daily basis, five days a week, for 5-7 days a week. For patients with cancer on a limited stage, radiation therapy is given two times in a day, five day in a week for 3 weeks. Unlike Chemotherapy, which is body-wide or systematic treatment, radiation is only administered to body areas affected by cancer. As a local treatment, side effects only happen on the body area which undergoes such treatment.

Chest radiation –According to some studies involving patients with small, limited-stage cancer of the lungs cell, chest radiation has the capability to decreases the possibility of cancer (in the chest) reoccurrence after an initial treatment. In addition, radiation improves the chance of curing the cancer.

Radiation Therapy and Chemotherapy is what we called concurrent therapy, or the administration of both therapy at the same time. But in case of disease on the chest, radiation will be given after the completion of the chemotherapy, this process is called a sequential therapy. Sequential therapy are recommended or given to patients who have nearly severe tumor condition with large tumor or for those who are already sick even before they are diagnosed with cancer.

Chest radiation can also be used to patients with extensive-stage small cell lung cancer but shows a good response to the initial chemotherapy and still have disease in their lymph nodes or on their lungs.

Once radiation is administered concurrently, side effects of the two treatment are typically more pronounced. The good news is that benefits are also bigger in number compared to a treatment done sequentially.

Chest radiation side effects commonly occur and experienced after few weeks of the treatment. Some of which are mild reddening of the skin on the back and chest, fatigue, and painful or difficult swallowing because of inflammation on the esophagitis (inner lining of esophagus). The latter symptom is carefully monitored and can be cured with the right pain medications.

However, long term side effects can also possibly occur and can be observed months after the completion of the radiation therapy. This may include scarring and/or inflammation of the patient's normal lung which surrounds the cancer which is also known as pneumonitis. Patients with pneumonitis will experience shortness in breathing, coughing and increased production of sputum.

Effectiveness of Small Cell Lung Cancer Treatment

Chemotherapy is undeniably beneficial to patients with any sorts of cancer, particularly those who have small cell lung cancer. A number of patients who undergo on such medications have improved both the duration and rate or survival and the quality of their life. Before the invention of chemotherapy, or even now if calculated, patients who are suffering from small cell lung cancer can survive only within weeks.

Even though this disease can be considered an aggressive one, it is still responsive to an initial chemotherapy as well as radiation. The treatment goal for patients with limited-stage disease is cure which is successfully achieved in 20-25% of patients.

 Patients who are suffering from limited-stage disease are highly responsive to radiotherapy and chemotherapy together, with substantial shrinkage of tumor noted in 80-100% of patients. Approximately half of these patients portray complete response without any remaining indication of the cancer. Unluckily, most patients are still pone to recurrence of cancer that becomes more resistant to a subsequent treatment.

In cases of extensive-stage disease, chemotherapy or radiation therapy can never deliver complete cure. This treatment can only maintain the quality of patient's life, prolong their survival and relieve painful symptoms. Although it can't totally cure the disease, these treatments, specifically chemotherapy offers higher response rate with 10-15% of whom achieve complete response while 60-80% of them having substantial tumor shrinkage.

In spite of favorable results brought by these treatments, most patient still experience recurrence or relapse of the said disease just within 1 to 2 years. If the kind of chemotherapy given to the recurrence cancer is not effective anymore, a different type of the same treatment will be given to provide some symptom relief and modest survival improvement.

Smoking Cessation

Smoking cigars, cigarettes or pipes is the typical cause of a lung cancer. In fact, cigarettes smoking have been indicated as the cause of approximately 400,000 deaths in United States. Furthermore, second-hand smoke exposure is projected to cause around 40, 000 deaths annually.

Quitting smoking is of significant importance if you want to be cured. Just because you just have limited-stage disease, you are already allowed to continue smoking. Well, it's all at your own risk. Patients who never quite smoking are less likely to experience improvements even though they already undergo into required treatment.

This is possibly because after their first cancer survival, they never quit smoking which results on developing of another lung cancer. Quitting smoking is not just important in prevention of cancer recurrence, it is also important to avoid further damage or disease caused by frequent chemotherapy, surgery and radiation therapy.

Getting away from cigarettes may be a hard task, especially because these are really addictive. But this is never an impossible thing to accomplish. With determination and self-discipline, sooner or later you can live normal life again without relying on cigarettes

To completely get cured from lung treatment, it will be best to have a comprehensive knowledge of he proper lung function before and after receiving any of the said treatment. Generally, patients are recommended to stop quitting.

Brain Radiation and Role of Surgery in Small Cell Lung Cancer

Brain Radiation – The brain of an individual suffering from limited-stage spread cell lung cancer is commonly prone to a tumor spread, also known as metastasis. For patients with both extensive-stage and limited-stage disease whose brain scans shows normal brain structure are still recommended to take radiation treatment after their initial treatment which may include chemotherapy and radiation or just plain chemotherapy to prevent or substantially reduces chances of developing tumor spread and prolong survival.

The preventive radiation therapy is known in clinical term as PCI or prophylactic cranial irradiation. This is often recommended to individuals whose body has shown partial or complete response to the primary chemoradiotherapy or chemotherapy.

Through the use of modern techniques, prophylactic cranial irradiation causes tolerable level of side effects that will not last long. This includes fatigue, hair loss, and itching and redness of scalp which typically improves after few weeks or even months after undergoing PCI.

There are also some uncommon long-term effects including intellectual and neurologic difficulties such as difficulty in concentrating, loss of short-term memory, and even instability in walking. This side effects are commonly experienced by elderly patients who undergo PCI, thus the benefits and risks of this treatment should be cautiously considered especially for patients over 70 years of age who already suffers from neurological problems. In case PCI are required, long term side effects can still be reduced through administering chemotherapy and PCI at different times.

The Role of Surgery in Small Cell Lung Cancer

The duration and probability of patient's survival cannot be determined by any surgery. Considering the speed of small cell lung cancer, undergoing surgery which aims to remove lung tumor can never give an assurance that the patient has greater level of survival. But this doesn't mean it is generally useless.

Few of cancer patients, typically less than 5%, whose cancer are detected on its earliest stage can still acquire benefits from a surgery. For this patients, if a surgery is followed by a chemotherapy, the survival duration can reach up to 5 years with a survival rate up to 35-40%.

Surgery can be beneficial for patients who show no evidence of cancer spread on the lymph nodes or in other area of the body but has single tumor that is confined to lungs' one lobe. In this case a mediastinoscopy (procedure commonly performed by thoracic surgeon) is considered first before the surgery.

This procedure involves a thin tube or scope which is inserted on the sternum (skin above the patient's breast bone), and to the mediastinum (the chest's middle part between the left and right lungs). The tube will be used to withdraw or get a sample tissue, typically a lymph node. Afterwards the sample tissue will be assesses through using a microscope in order to determine whether or not there is a cancer cell.

In case there is no sign or presence of cancer cells on the lymph nodes, surgical removal of lung cancer which is followed by a chemotherapy or chemoradiotheraphy will be a reasonable treatment for the disease.

High risk of nutritional supplements

An estimated 65% to 85% of cancer patients use supplements. Some vitamins, minerals, herbs, amino acids and antioxidants interfere with how well cancer drugs work or block them from working at all and drastically increase the rate of failure. Some dietary supplements can cause sensitivity and severe reactions when taken during chemotherapy and radiation treatments also.

Many supplements cause cancer to grow as a secondary action and that is why most supplements should be avoided in any cancer treatment and you should focus on a healthy diet and herbs and only vitamins that have extensive clinical data if you are deficient.

Vitamins cannot be isolated from their complexes and still perform their specific life functions within the cells. When isolated into artificial commercial forms, like ascorbic acid, these purified synthetics act as drugs in the body. They are no longer vitamins, and to call them such is inaccurate. - Dr. Tim O'Shea

Example: In 50% of people the amino acid L-Arginine kills cancer, in the other 50% makes it grow much faster. Some vitamins interfere with hormones and can trigger the cancer to grow faster.

So no supplements should be taken, everything should come from diet/food. Extreme Caution should be taken with any vitamin, amino acid, mineral and or herb. Some vitamins are considered very safe for Cancer but can cause a problem with Chemotherapy or herbs taken. Please be very careful.

Vitamin E supplements are shown in studies to increase the size and speed of Lung cancer and tumor growth, but in dietary intake of Vitamin E it slows it down. The issue is most Vitamins only have one part of the entire vitamin and not the entire vitamin, without the balance it causes a side effect.

The only vitamin that has been shown to fight Small Cell Lung Cancer in a vitamin form is Vitamin D, again it should be taken with Curcumin because it selectively binds with Curcumin as it activates Vitamin D receptors to switch the immune system on to fight your cancer. Vitamin D can also be created from going out in the sun, the problem is as you get older your body creates less Vitamin D while being in the sun. Estrogen is said to fuel lung cancer, Vitamin D is a steroid Vitamin and Curcumin has steroid affects which reduce estrogen, block it and increase testosterone to kill the small cell lung cancer.

Alkaline the Body and increase oxygen levels

It is not recommended for small cell cancers because though it does work, it can cause the cancer to grow much quicker and is a very delicate balancing act that kills more people than are successful because it causes faster growth. Please read on to understand as diet can also cause this to happen.

Please Note: Eating more alkaline foods helps shift your body's pH and oxygenate your system. But also makes cancer grow faster if not counter balanced very delicately.

Note of Caution:

Cancer seems to grow slowly in a high acid environment (the acids cause it to partially destroy itself) and may actually grow more quickly as your body becomes more alkaline prior to reaching the healthy pH. Which means reaching slightly above 7.4 where the cancer becomes close to dormant at 8 and over 8 when it dies.

This is why you must counteract this process until your body gets a higher PH with Curcumin, Milk Thistle, ECGC,Q10, and/or K2 alone or in combination or any other drug that stops the growth of cancer. My Opinon as the best is Curcumin as a must or combination.

If you wish to Alkaline the body use Sodium Bicarbonate (arm and hammer baking soda), yes it is safe to take and does not interfere with chemo or any other by product in the body. Bicarbonate is in every cell and body fluid in the body and sodium is not only a protector of organs it is used for excretion of toxins in the body and to increase overall PH.

Cancer is acidic and Baking Soda is Alkaline, so it destroys cancer by changing its environment but it does have complications even though it is a wonderful medical drug used in every Emergency Room in America. Sodium bicarbonate cancer treatment focuses on delivering natural chemotherapy in a way that effectively kills cancer cells while dramatically reducing the brutal side effects and costs experienced with standard chemotherapy treatments.

Oncologists do understand that bicarbonate is necessary to protect their patients from the toxicity and harm done by highly toxic chemicals used in chemotherapy. They also know it is extraordinarily helpful to patients receiving radiation treatments in protecting the kidneys and other tissues of the body from radioactive damages. So most chemotherapy treatments include sodium bicarbonate mixed or pre-injected into patients before or during treatment.

This year these same researchers reported that bicarbonate increases tumor pH (i.e., make it more alkaline) and also inhibits spontaneous metastases (Robey 2009). They showed that oral sodium bicarbonate increased the pH of tumors and also reduced the formation of spontaneous metastases.

I have seen it work on an unresponsive patient with 70 years old that was in a complete vegetable state recover cognition fully within 12 hrs with just one teaspoon of baking soda with a glucose delivery system such as stated below.

How Much is Safe and how:

Bicarbonate with Black Strap molasses fulfills the role of the glucose."Sodium bicarbonate therapy is harmless, fast and effective because it is extremely diffusible. A therapy with bicarbonate for cancer should be set up with strong dosage, continuously, and with pauseless cycles in a destruction work which should proceed from the beginning to the end without interruption for at least 7-8 days. In general a mass of 2-3-4 centimeters will begin to consistently regress from the third to the fourth day, and collapses from the fourth to the fifth," says Dr Simoncini. Sodium bicarbonate can be used orally in doses of 1/ 2 tsp in 4 oz of water every two hours for pain relief as well as gastrointestinal upset, not to exceed 7 doses per day.

Here are the exact instructions for oral use from the Arm and Hammer baking soda package. Directions: Add 1/ 2 teaspoon to 1/ 2 glass (4 fl. oz.) of water every 2 hours, or as directed by physician. Dissolve completely in water.
Accurately measure 1/ 2 teaspoon.

Do not take more than the following amounts in 24 hours:

--Seven 1/ 2 teaspoons.

--Three 1/ 2 teaspoons if you are over 60 years.

Do not use the maximum dosage for more than 2 weeks.

Other Information: Each 1/ 2 teaspoon contains 616 mg sodium.

1 teaspoon of baking soda with 1 teaspoon of Black Strap molasses and one cup of water. Not warmed or heated water, Just room temperature.

Warning and Pre-existing Conditions:

Overly aggressive therapy with Sodium Bicarbonate Injection, USP can result in metabolic alkalosis (associated with muscular twitchings, irritability, and tetany) and hypernatremia. Caution should also be maintained when pushing oral dosages up to the maximum levels suggested for oral administration as well.

For people with the rare illnesses of Bartter syndrome or Gitelman syndrome, bicarbonate may be contraindicated. These rare sufferers may add a few drops of Real-Lemon juice concentrate to any bicarbonate-containing beverage to neutralize it. Serious precautions should be taken by individuals who suffer from chronic pulmonary problems. If a person has significant lung disease, their brain shifts to breathing in response to a lowered O2 level so it won't respond to the accumulating CO2.

Extra caution: needs to be taken with cancer patients with severe heart, renal, and hepatic problems. Dr. Simoncini says, "In any case, however, it is best to try to reach the maximum tolerable quantity, as a dosage that is too low or too thinly distributed over time cannot be effective in depth. In some patients, although not afflicted by other pathological conditions other than a tumor, if there are many masses or the masses have large dimensions we have sometimes observed a remarkable increase in the temperature up to 39 degrees centigrade in the first days of therapy with bicarbonate. This is the effect of the brutal lysis of the colonies, which in some cases is even responsible for the high amylaceous contents and for transitory renal insufficiency sometimes associated with a bladder urinary block which can be solved through catheterization. Hypertension or hypotension events as well as episodes of relapsing cephalea complete the picture of side effects which, it is wise to emphasize, are rare and brief. That is without negative after effects."

Sodium bicarbonate is safe when taken with appropriate caution and knowledge, extremely inexpensive and effective when it comes to reducing cancer tissues. It's an irresistible chemical, cyanide to cancer cells for it hits the cancer cells with a shock wave of alkalinity, which allows much more oxygen into the cancer cells than they can tolerate. Cancer cells do not survive well in the presence of higher levels of oxygen. Sircus, Mark (2010-06-03). Sodium Bicarbonate - Full Medical Review Medical Veritas Association.

High-Dose Intravenous Vitamin C up to 150,000mg 1-2 times per week:

In many cancers it can cure and kill the cancer completly (NSCC) but in every single study involving(SCC) small cell lung cancer, it has been shown to only increase life span and help symptomes and not cure. More studies are needed in order to prove or disprove but at this time for SCLC it does not seem to show it as beneficial or a negative, other than making the cancer side effects better. Please note oral Vitamin C does not work at all but can make symptoms better.

Also, Treatment averages $1600-2000 per month and if stopped abruptly can cause scurvy. Similar effects are shown with I.V. HYDROGEN PEROXIDE but cause a lot more damage than good.

Intravenous Curcumin has been shown to work in all cancers and increased success by 50% if white light is added to the cancer treatment directly to the tumor. Problem is very few places in the United States do this treatment. It also has no effect if stopped abruptly.

Hyperthermia Cancer Treatment also called thermal therapy or thermotherapy

This treatment works and has been studied for years but is expensive and can be dangerous if done by the wrong person. They heat either your body, blood or the tumor directly to temperatures between 106 and 110 F. Most normal tissues are not damaged during hyperthermia if the temperature remains under 111°F. The treatment cost can vary from $1,500-20,000 but this takes us to another point. At 95 F your body starts to spread and grow cancer so use of sauna, steam room and/ or a biomat which is infrared pad cost $500-1500 can all maintain a healthy temperature of your body of a minimum of 98 F. Heat repairs the body, it balances fluids and it activates toxin cell death to cancer and any other bacteria and/or infection.

Please Note: Cancer is said to start spreading at 95 F so keep a thermometer handy and check your temperature regularly. This along with PH strips, cancer PH is around 4.5 so try to eat more green vegetables, apples and a healthy diet to increase the PH levels.

IMPORTANT NOTICE: These treatments are synergistic meaning they work alone as well as together, if together dosage must be reduced to half since most do a lot of the same things. People that are diabetic, have high blood pressure and/or other medical problems should further investigate interactions between prescribed medication and or sickness with agents below before starting any new medical regiment.

If you are planning on Chemotherapy. Milk Thistle and Curcumin reverse possible drug resistance and make cancer cells more sensitive to chemotherapy. Take these two for at least a week before chemotherapy to increase the chances of success.   Always consult with your oncologist before starting any program.

The 6 Agents that have proven to Destroy Small Cell Cancer

The 6 Agents that have proven to Destroy Small Cell Cancer

1. Curcumin (Tumeric) Changes Regulation of DNA and Reprograms it to kill Cancer.
*Curcumin is the only thing on earth that physically binds to as many as 33 different proteins, there are more than 40 biomolecules that are involved in cell death induced by curcumin on cancer. If is safe to use with Chemotherapy and not only makes chemotherapy stronger it protects healthy cells from damage because of Chemotherapy. Curcumin induces autophagy which is when cancer cells eat themselves, it also shrinks tumors, stops the spread of tumors, stops Angiogenesis Stops and reverses Cachexia, stops the fermentation process, removes cancer drug resistance, removes lactic acid, alkalizes the body, increases cellular oxygen, Survival Signal Deactivation, Removes side effects of cancer- Loss of hunger, energy levels, Anti-inflammatory, constipation and pain. Half-life is 1 to 4 hours. Absorption is very low unless taken with Bioprine (Pepper Extract) or BCM-95 which can stay in the blood for 8 hrs. Full Explanation under product spotlight page 13. **If you can find a Clinic (Naturalpathy, Internal Medicine) that does Curcumin iv, I would seriously look at getting treatment done. There are a few places in the United States that do it. If you search online for naturopathic IV curcumin***

or Intravenous Curcumin + your state or Your State + IV curcumin or same as rest but replace IV with intravenous : you should find some in Georgia, Colorado, Arizona, Florida, BC Canada and many European Countries.

2. ECGC

EGCG It is safe to use with Chemotherapy and not only makes chemotherapy stronger it protects healthy cells from damage because of Chemotherapy. It inhibits and shrinks tumor growth, invasion, angiogenesis and metastasis, Stops and reverses Cachexia, removes cancer drug resistance, removes lactic acid, alkalizes the body, increases cellular oxygen, Removes side effects of cancer- energy levels, Anti-inflammatory, constipation and pain.

3. Coenzyme Q10 (Only take Ubiquinol(The active part of Q10)

Coenzyme Q10 , To start off 90% or more of all cancer patients have a Q10 deficiency. Cancer starts by changing the DNA inside cells and make it reproduce, one of the amazing things Q10 does is restore a cancer cell's ability to kill itself when it cannot in rare cancers, while not impacting normal cells. Q10 is involved in energy production in the body it stops Cachexia. It removes efficiency of radiation therapy, should not be used with chemotherapy. Some Findings show that supplementation with coQ10 can cause complete regression of tumors in advanced small cell lung cancer. For best results add Curcumin which is a natural "cancer killer" and CoQ10 is a cell energizer at the molecular level.

4. Vitamin K2 (menaquinone)also known as MK4

Vitamin K induces apoptosis through activation of a "suicide protein. "Clinical trials of newer chemotherapy agents have shown that when chemotherapy no longer works vitamin K being added to makes it rapidly suppress growth in all lung cancer cell lines tested. Vitamin K's activity also activates "oncosis," a form of stress-activated cell death to which tumor cells are particularly susceptible. Because of their high growth rate, tumor cells consume vast amounts of glucose. And because they can rapidly outgrow their blood supplies, that high metabolism means they use up oxygen rapidly, making them especially vulnerable to oxidant stress—much more so than the healthy tissues around them. Vitamin K targets tumor cells for destruction by stimulating oxidative stress, without toxicity to healthy tissues. Another unique mechanism is autophagy, in which cancer cells essentially "eat" themselves by releasing their own digestive enzymes internally.

5. Milk Thistle (Silymarin)

Silymarin works like chemotherapy without killing good cells. It is shown to stop cancer cells from dividing and reproducing, shortening the lifespan of cancer cells. Reduce blood supply to tumors, cause adoposis, reverse drug resistance to chemotherapy and provides antioxidant support for chemotherapy while making it more efficient.

6. *Ganoderma lucidum-(reishi)*

G. lucidum kills drug-sensitive small-cell lung cancer, drug-resistant small-cell lung cancer, and normal lung cancer cells. The researchers discovered that G. lucidum killed lung cancer cells the same way as chemotherapy without becoming resistant and without killing good cells. It also restored the immune system and super-activated it, while improving overall well being. It is tumor suppressant and inhibits tumors from spreading.

The 6 Agents of Small Cell Cancer individual Studies.
There are thousands of studies on each ingredient that you may find but below are the most targeted to get you started.

Curcumin (Tumeric) BEST SMALL CELL CANCER TREATMENT IN THE WORLD.

Curcumin can impact all of these areas because they are all affected by a transcription factor (something in the cell that binds to DNA) called Nuclear Factor kappa B (or NFkB for short). The picture below shows the various signaling molecules that NFkB impacts which cause the growth and ultimately the metastasis of a tumor:

NFκB

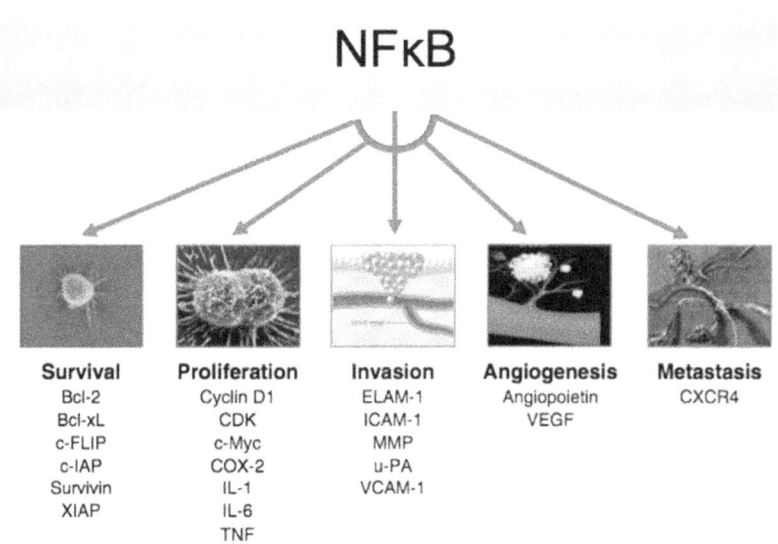

Survival	Proliferation	Invasion	Angiogenesis	Metastasis
Bcl-2	Cyclin D1	ELAM-1	Angiopoietin	CXCR4
Bcl-xL	CDK	ICAM-1	VEGF	
c-FLIP	c-Myc	MMP		
c-IAP	COX-2	u-PA		
Survivin	IL-1	VCAM-1		
XIAP	IL-6			
	TNF			

Curcumin inhibits NFkB, and is thus able to greatly impact cancer progression. Take a look at this CAT scan from a patient with liver cancer who had already failed chemotherapy

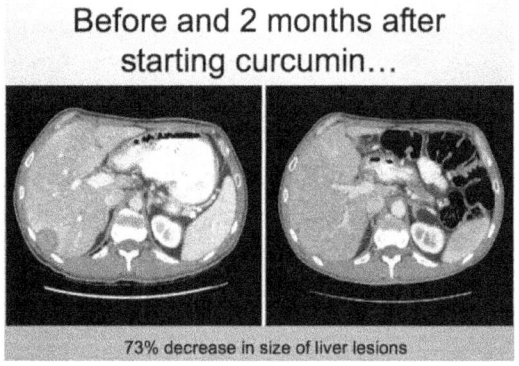

Before and 2 months after starting curcumin…

73% decrease in size of liver lesions

Dillon N, Aggarwal BB, Kurzrock R. Phase II Trial of Curcumin in Patients With Advanced Pancreatic Cancer Clin Cancer Res 2008; 14(14) July 15, 2008
http://www.ncbi.nlm.nih.gov/pubmed/18628464
The patient who's CAT scan you see above had to take 8 grams (not milligrams) a day, which is 8,000 mg.

Curcumin blocks *small cell lung cancer* cells migration (spread), invasion, angiogenesis, cell cycle and neoplasia. *Curcumin* induces *small cell lung cancer* NCI-H446 cell apoptosis via the reactive oxygen species-mediated mitochondrial pathway. Prevent the formation of cancerous cells.

Curcumin is inherently non-toxic. A team of researchers led by Dr. Ajay Goel at the Baylor

University Medical Center in Dallas, Texas have found that even 10,000 to 12,000 mg per day can be taken with few or no side effects. Since many people who have cancer have problems with swallowing or with various kinds of indigestion, they recommend a liposome form of the supplement so their patients don't have to take as many capsules to get the same amount of active curcumin.

Scientists at the Laoining Cancer Institute in Shenyang in the People's Republic of China have found that curcumin stops the proliferation of single small cell lung cancer cells into masses of small cell lung cancer cells. It does this by inhibiting an enzymatic process known as STAT3 phosphorylation.If the cancer cells have already proliferated, then curcumin inhibits the ability of the mass of cells to adhere to each other as a colony. Curcumin does this by interfering with the production of three proteins known as Bcl-(X)L, cyclin B1, and survivin. If the cancer cells have survived long enough to reproduce themselves and form a tumor, then curcumin interferes with their ability to use the proteins ICAM-1, MMP-2, MMP-7, and VEGF to invade surrounding healthy tissues. And if the cancer tumor has spread into nearby healthy tissue, then curcumin stops the production of another chemical called IL-6, which helps the tumor establish its own blood supply through a process called angiogenesis.

For people with small cell lung cancer who continue to smoke, curcumin deactivates the "survival signal" that nicotine sends to the cancer cells. This "survival signal," as researchers call it, refers to the survival of the cancer, not the survival of the patient. This signal reduces the survivor of the smoker.Not everyone who has cancer and smokes gets worse as a result of smoking. That depends on the action of a gene called p53. If the smoker has a variant of this cancer-destructive gene that isn't deactivated by smoking, then smoking doesn't make the cancer worse.

If the cancer cells have already proliferated, then curcumin inhibits the ability of the mass of cells to adhere to each other as a colony. Curcumin does this by interfering with the production of three proteins known as Bcl-(X)L, cyclin B1, and survivin. If the cancer cells have survived long enough to reproduce themselves and form a tumor, then curcumin interferes with their ability to use the proteins ICAM-1, MMP-2, MMP-7, and VEGF to invade surrounding healthy tissues. And if the cancer tumor has spread into nearby healthy tissue, then curcumin stops the production of another chemical called IL-6, which helps the tumor establish its own blood supply through a process called angiogenesis.

Curcumin has a diverse range of molecular targets, supporting the concept that it acts upon numerous biochemical and molecular cascades. Curcumin physically binds to as many as 33 different proteins, including thioredoxin reductase, cyclooxygenase-2, (COX2), protein kinase C, 5-lipoxygenase (5-LOX), and tubulin. Various molecular targets modulated by this agent include transcription factors, growth factors and their receptors, cytokines, enzymes, and genes regulating cell proliferation, and apoptosis. Curcumin has been shown to inhibit the proliferation and survival of almost all types of tumor cells. Accumulating evidence suggests that the mode of curcumin-induced cell death is mediated both by the activation of cell death pathways and by the inhibition of growth/proliferation pathways. Many studies indicate the selective role of curcumin towards cancer cells than normal cells. We could identify more than 40 biomolecules that are involved in cell death induced by curcumin .The mechanistic relationship among different signal transduction pathways, whether acting alone or together, leading to apoptosis is described. Because curcumin mediates its effect through multiple cell signaling pathways, the likelihood of developing resistance to it is less. How these interrelated pathways are activated is explained below.

ECGC
The green tea polyphenol, epigallocatechin-3-gallate inhibits telomerase and induces apoptosis in drug-resistant lung cancer cells.

Epidemiological studies on humans and investigations in animal models suggest that consumption of green tea has anti-cancer effects. Small-cell lung carcinoma (SCLC) has a poor prognosis, particularly due to the development of drug resistance. We investigated the effects of the green tea polyphenol, epigallocatechin-3-gallate (EGCG) on human SCLC cells. EGCG had similar effects (IC(50) of approximately 70 microM) on drug-sensitive (H69) and drug-resistant (H69VP) SCLC cells, indicating that it is not part of the drug resistance phenotype expressed in these cells. In both cell lines, incubation in EGCG at 1 x IC(50) for 24h resulted in 50-60% reduced telomerase activity as measured by a PCR-based assay for telomeric repeats. Colorimetric assays of cells treated for 36 h with EGCG demonstrated a reduction in activities of caspases 3 (50%) and 9 (70%) but not caspase 8, indicating initiation of apoptosis. DNA fragmentation as measured by ELISA occurred within cells treated with EGCG and this was confirmed by TUNEL staining. Flow cytometric analysis of SCLC cells incubated for 36 h in EGCG indicated a cell-cycle block in S phase. These data indicate the potential use of EGCG, and possibly green tea, in treating SCLC.

Although EGCG has been tested in numerous cancer cell lines and some clinical trials, there are minimal data on its effectiveness in lung cancer. It seems that EGCG does impair growth in small cell lung cancer cells, but has a variable effect on the limited number of NSCLC cell lines tested (24, 25). The evidence that tea polyphenols exert inhibitory effects in numerous and distinct cancer cells led us to investigate the activity of these compounds on NSCLC cells *in vitro* and *in vivo* to determine if EGCG in combination with targeting strategies would be more effective than treatment with single agents. In this report, we show the effectiveness of EGCG to sensitize previously insensitive NSCLC cell lines to erlotinib *in vitro* and *in vivo*.

Sadava, D et al., The Green Tea Polyphenol, Epigallocatechin-3-Gallate Inhibits Telomerase and Induces Apoptosis in Drug-Resistant Lung Cancer Cells. Biochemical and Biophysical Research Communications, 2007 Jun 14;

Less than 24 hours after introducing EGCG to the tumor cells, we saw a 50-60 percent reduction in telomerase activity,". "That reduction resulted in a number of the hallmarks of programmed cell death: the cancer cells' DNA started breaking, the cells stopped dividing, and the production of an enzyme [caspase] that destroys cells' nuclei was induced.

Coenzyme Q10 (Ubiquinol)

The survival rate for the study period was one hundred percent (four deaths were expected). Six patients were reported to show some evidence of remission; however, incomplete clinical data were provided, and information suggestive of remission was presented for only three of the six patients.

None of the six patients had evidence of further metastases. For all 32 patients, decreased use of painkillers, improved quality of life, and an absence of weight loss were reported. Whether painkiller use and quality of life were measured objectively (e.g., from pharmacy records and validated questionnaires, respectively) or subjectively (from patient self-reports) was not specified.

In a follow-up study, one of the six patients with a reported remission and a new patient were treated for several months with higher doses of coenzyme Q10 (390 and 300 milligrams per day, respectively).[29] Surgical removal of the primary breast tumor in both patients had been incomplete.

After 3 to 4 months of high-level coenzyme Q10 supplementation, both patients appeared to experience complete regression of their residual breast tumors (assessed by clinical examination and mammography). It should be noted that a different patient identifier was used in the follow-up study for the patient who had participated in the original study. Studies on other Small-cell cancers have also shown the same.

"In late 1993, Dr. Folkers arranged for the first clinical trial of Co Q10 at a clinic in Copenhagen, Denmark. Doctors treated 32 patients with advanced, "high risk" breast cancer. In addition to appropriate surgery and conventional treatment, each patient was given 90 mg of CoQ10 per day. They also received other vitamins, minerals, antioxidants, and essential fatty acids. On this regimen, 6 of the 32 patients showed partial tumor regressions, significant in "advanced" patients. Then in October 1993, a strange thing happened: one of these six women, on her own, increased her dosage from 90 to 390 mg per day. By the next month, her doctors wrote, "the tumor was no longer palpable and in the following month, a mammogram confirmed the disappearance of her tumor. After that, another woman in the group also increased her dose, this time to 300 mg. Her tumor also soon disappeared and a clinical examination revealed no evidence of the prior residual tumor, nor of distant metastases

Vitamin K2 (menaquinone)also known as MK4

In several different types of lung cancer, including small cell, squamous cell, and adenocarcinomas, vitamin K induces apoptosis through activation of a "suicide protein. Finally, three of vitamin K's synergistic anticancer mechanisms have recently been identified. Vitamin K3 inhibits DNA-building enzymes.22 Vitamins K2 and K3 *block* new blood vessel formation essential to support the rapid growth of tumor tissue.22-24 And vitamin K3 disrupts crucial intracellular communications networks composed of microtubules, preventing the cells from proliferating in a coordinated fashion.25. Vitamin K2 also induces MDS cells to differentiate into healthy white blood cells. 90 mg/day of MK4 MK4 with dosages ranging from 10 mg/day up to135 mg/day orally (83% received an oral dose of 45 mg/day). Improvements began within 1 to 3 months. They concluded that MK4 was a successful treatment in reducing cancer cell numbers in 71.4% of the patients. The data was strongly encouraging for elderly patients who couldn't tolerate intensive chemotherapy or stem cell transplantation and indicates that VK2 was chemopreventive against leukemia.

Vitamin K2 (menaquinone-4: VK2) has been reported to show apoptosis and differentiation-inducing effects on leukemia cells. Furthermore, the clinical benefits of using VK2 have been demonstrated for the treatment of the patients with acute leukemia and myelodysplastic syndromes. In the present study, we examined the in vitro effects of VK2 on lung carcinoma cell lines LU-139 and LU-130 for small cell carcinomas, PC-14 and CCL-185 for adenocarcinomas, LC-AI and LC-1/sq for squamous cell carcinomas, and IA-LM for large cell carcinoma, respectively. Treatment with VK2 for 48 to 96 h resulted in cell growth suppression in a dose-dependent manner in all cell lines tested. IC50 (50% inhibitory concentration) for VK2 ranged from 7.5 to 75 micro M, and there was no relation between the efficacy of growth suppression by VK2 and tissue type of lung carcinoma cell lines. Morphologic features of the cells treated with VK2 were typical for apoptosis along with caspase-3 activation and becoming positive for APO2.7 monoclonal antibody, an antibody which specifically detects the cell undergoing apoptosis. In addition to the leukemia cell line, LU-139 cells accumulated into G0/G1 phase during 72-h exposure to VK2. Combined treatment of cisplatin plus VK2 resulted in enhanced cytocidal effect compared to the cells treated with either cisplatin or VK2 alone. Since VK2 is a safe medicine without prominent adverse effects including bone marrow suppression, our data strongly suggest the therapeutic possibility of using VK2 for the treatment of patients with lung carcinoma.

Milk Thistle (Silymarin) -
Small cell lung *cancer* develops resistance to common chemotherapies milk thistle Reversed drug-resistantance in small cell lung cancer. (Stops cell signaling and can cause adoposis p53 activvation/cell cycle arrest) Milk thistle is often prescribed by to protect from the hepatoxic effects of chemotherapy drugs. Silymarin modulates imbalance between cell survival and apoptosis through interference with the expressions of cell cycle regulators and proteins involved in apoptosis. In addition, silymarin also showed anti-inflammatory as well as anti-metastatic activity.

Multitarget therapy of cancer by Silymarin
Silymarin, a flavonolignan from milk thistle (Silybum marianum) plant, is used for the protection against various liver conditions in both clinical settings and experimental models. In this review, we summarize the recent investigations and mechanistic studies regarding possible molecular targets of silymarin for cancer prevention. Number of studies has established the cancer chemopreventive role of silymarin in both *in vivo* and *in vitro* models. Silymarin modulates imbalance between cell survival and apoptosis through interference with the expressions of cell

cycle regulators and proteins involved in apoptosis. In addition, silymarin also showed anti-inflammatory as well as anti-metastatic activity. Further, the protective effects of silymarin and its major active constituent, silibinin, studied in various tissues, suggest a clinical application in cancer patients as an adjunct to establibled therapies, to prevent or reduce chemotherapy as well as radiotherapy-induced toxicity. This review focuses on the chemistry and analogues of silymarin, multiple possible molecular mechanisms, *in vitro* as well as *in vivo* anticancer activities, and studies on human clinical trials.

The dose of silymarin used in studies has ranged from 200 to 800 mg per day.

Ganoderma lucidum-(reishi)

Research published in Cancer letters1 highlights the benefits Red Reishi (Ganoderma lucidum), as a complementary cancer treatment. Red Reishi has previously been studied for its effects on leukaemia, as well as on cancers of the breast, bladder, colon, and prostate, but the new study set out to investigate its effects on small-cell lung cancer and took extracts of G. lucidum which were tested on three different types of cells: drug-sensitive small-cell lung cancer, drug-resistant small-cell lung cancer, and normal lung cells.

The researchers discovered that G. lucidum killed lung cancer cells as they responded to the herb much in the same way as they would react to chemotherapy drugs. Yet unlike chemotherapy drugs, which can also be toxic to healthy cells, herbal extracts were more deadly to cancer cells than to normal cells, indicating that they have some ability to specifically target cancer.

Dosage
Traditional practitioners recommend 0.5 to 1 g daily, 2 to 5 g daily for chronic illness, and up to G. lucidum **15 g extract daily for serious illness**. 5 The Chinese pharmacopoeia recommends 6 to 12 g extract daily. 5 Doses up to Ganopoly 5.4 g daily (equivalent to 81 g of the fruiting body) for 12 weeks have been used in clinical trials.

Adverse Reactions
Reported adverse reactions from reishi include dizziness, dry mouth, stomach upset, nosebleed, bone pain, skin irritation, diarrhea, and constipation. 2 , 31

In a small, placebo-controlled trial designed to determine adverse reactions related to reishi use, 4 g of extract daily for 10 days taken by healthy adults resulted in no differences between participants receiving reishi and those taking placebo. 48 No changes in blood CD4, CD8, or CD19 were observed, and insignificant increases in CD56 were noted.

Toxicology
Research reveals little information regarding toxicity with the use of reishi mushroom. A mean lethal dose has been estimated to be 10 to 21 g per kg body weight. Animal experiments have tested dosages up to 38 g/kg

How to Take (recommended dosage, active amounts, other details)

The standard dose of *Ganoderma lucidum* depends on the form of the supplement. A general *Ganoderma lucidum* extract does not separate the triterpenoids and the polysaccharides present in the mushroom, which make up the ethanolic and water-soluble extracts, respectively. The standard dose for the basic extract is 1.44g – 5.2g. The most popular dose is 5.2g, taken in three doses of 1,800mg.

The standard dosage for the ethanolic extract is 6mg. The water-soluble extract should be dosed similarly to the basic extract. The basic extract is essentially dehydrated mushroom powder, which makes it about 10 times as potent as the actual mushroom. This means that 5g of extract is similar to about 50g of whole mushroom.

Product Spotlight

Natural Medicine works the problem is understanding correct dosing and purity, it is hard to find or simply hard to understand to reproduce results from medical studies.

PLEASE NOTE:

Remember Pure extract is used in all scientific experiments so when shopping for herbs you must look for extract standardized amounts of active ingredient, below is the best of each.

Curcumin (Tumeric)

Important Notice: Oral curcumin is poorly absorbed from the bowel. There are multiple types of Curcumin including: Curcumin, Curcumin with Bioprine(Pepper) which is normally called Sabinsa or C3 complex, Theracurmin , Meriva, Longvida and BCM-95.All testing will show you different levels of absorption but clinical studies don't lie as easy.Longvida---Alzheimer's patients,Regeneration of Brain Stem Cells. Not for Cancer. Meriva and Theracurmin- Only metabolites, no anti-cancer activity

The best Curcumin available for Cancer is BCM-95 the second is Sabinsa which is also reffered to as C3 complex or Curcumin and Peperine.

• BCM-95® Curcumin has been proven to deliver up to 7 times more Curcumin into the bloodstream as the same amount of plain Curcumin. Studies Show BCM-95 has full anti-cancer activity and blocks all proteins and message transcription from cancer.

Life Extension Super Bio-curcumin, 400mg, Vegetarian Capsules, 60-Count
http://www.amazon.com/Life-Extension-Bio-curcumin-Vegetarian-Capsules/dp/B000X9P5GM/ref=sr_1_5?&ie=UTF8&qid=1438050736&sr=8-5&keywords=BCM95

$21.13 you will need 2-3 bottles a month.

Safe Dosage (Starting Dosage 1 pill x 3 times a day Same as taking 8,316mg a day every 6 hrs :1.5 bottles)

Caution: Never Start at Terminal dose, work your way up so your body can tolerate the treatment. Many people will not handle this dosage at first (Diarrhea, vomiting, stomach pains)

Always start off at Safe Dose above and then increase every week, so the body can adapt.

Terminal Dose (For Terminal Patients with less than 3 months to live- Highest dosage possible-2 pills x 3 times a day. Same as taking 16,632 mg day Every 6 hrs: 3 bottles a month

8,000-15,000 mg a day of normal curcumin/ BCM-95 can be cut down by 7x dosage because of high absorption levels. (Depending on body tolerance and how aggressive the cancer is.)

Curcumin is rapidly cleared from the blood (within 1-4 hours of ingestion, most of it is cleared. BCM-95 stays in the body over 8hrs) To maintain cancer killing effects in body , it is best to take it in divided doses throughout the day.

ECGC

NOW Foods EGCg, Green Tea Extract, 400mg, 180 Vcaps

200 total mg of pure EGCG. You need 1000-4000mg per day. 6-20 capsules per day
$15.75 you will need 1-4 bottles a month. (2 pills x 3 times day 1200mg ecgc 1 bottle month)

http://www.amazon.com/Foods-Green-Extract-400mg-Vcaps/dp/B001DNV5CA/ref=sr_1_1?ie=UTF8&qid=1437502410&sr=8-1&keywords=egcg

Coenzyme Q10

Life Extension Super Ubiquinol CoQ10 with Enhanced Mitochondrial, 100 Mg, Softgels, 60
$33.99 per bottle – 4-8 capsules daily (2-4 bottles a month)

http://www.amazon.com/Life-Extension-Ubiquinol-Enhanced-Mitochondrial/dp/B0010PK996/ref=sr_1_23?s=hpc&ie=UTF8&qid=1440183261&sr=1-23&keywords=ubiquinol

K2 Mk-4

Complementary Prescriptions - Ultra K2 15 mg 90 gels

Do not take this product if you are taking "blood thinners"
http://www.amazon.com/Complementary-Prescriptions-Ultra-K2-gels/dp/B0057ZGWDW/ref=sr_1_1?s=hpc&ie=UTF8&qid=1437499850&sr=1-1&keywords=Ultra+K2

http://www.cpmedical.net/ultra-k2.html

$36 per bottle -9 pills daily about 135mg - 3 bottles a month you will need

Silymarin/Milk Thistle

NOW Foods Silymarin/Milk Thistle 150mg, 120 Vcaps

2vcaps 300mg/ 240 of 80% silymarin (Up to 2-8 pills per day)

$11.99 per bottle 1-2 bottles per month you will need.

Ganoderma lucidum-(reishi)

*Mushroom extracts work not only directly cytostatic/ cytotoxic (i.e. killing cancer cells directly)
then also immunomodulatory (stimulating and orchestrating macrophages, lymphocytes, NK
cells and other parts of immune system to fight cancer. In every cancer case the essential
principle is to try to fight cancer at the such level that we kill tumor cells faster than they
multiply by tumor self division.*

*Single pharmaceutical compound PSP decreased cell survival at 20% , pointing out that
mushroom blends have stronger cytotoxic effects compared with the single compound. Look
Below for decreased cell survival at 80% in Myko san Agarikon.1 and Mykoprotect.1*

*NuSci Reishi Mushroom Extract Powder Standardized 30% Polysaccharides 500 grams (1.1 lb,
17.6 oz)*
$42.95 ($2.44 / oz) + $5.49 shipping you will need on average 2-3 bags a month

My Personal Opinion Strategy to Kill Small Cell Lung Cancer

All 5 of these agents activate and repair Cytotoxic T cells directly and indirectly.
This is a personal opinion on the most effective sequence to take the natural agents to be the
most effective without unexpected side effects that force the retardation of treatment. All work
together and can be taken separate, as you add steps reduce dose until your body accepts the
treatment without side effects and then you can start increasing dosages again.

PRE-STEP
ZINC

Stop, Reverse, destroy Cancer and Regain the Lost Sense of Taste
The p53 Adiposis/tumor suppressor is a transcription factor that contains a single zinc ion near its DNA binding interface, so without ZINC the body cannot kill cancer. Secondly, Hedgehog Pathway Activation is required in Small Cell Lung Cancer. Hedgehog pathway inhibition slows and stops the progression of disease and delay cancer recurrence in individuals with SCLC. Zinc will inhibit the production of the Hedgehog ligand, and therefore inhibit the Hedgehog pathway. Please refer to Zinc Very Important Document.

Special Note About Zinc:
The human body contains about 2000-3000 mg of Elemental zinc, of which about 2-3 mg are lost daily through kidneys, bowel, and sweat glands. The biologic half-life of zinc in the body is about 9 months, so it can take months or years for changes in dietary habits to substantially change zinc status, unless the intake is very high for short periods. 220 mg zinc sulfate Capsules: Each gives you about 50 mg of elemental zinc. Most people can tolerate 50 mg of elemental zinc or 1 tablet of 200mg zinc sulfate, you can also purchase pure elemental zinc. Please note, many people take up to 200-300 mg of elemental zinc per day when fighting cancer. Please check with your doctor before doing this.

Step 1
Curcumin

Why: full activation of every cancer pathway allows the body to reprogram it's self into a cancer killing machine. **If you don't take anything else in your fight against cancer, Curcumin is your go to medicine. Also, as stated above in The Curcumin section: If you can get IV treatment of Curcumin it is well worth it.**

Step 2
ECGC
Why: Removes the lactic acid build up, alkalizes the body and reverses cachexia, then it goes into increasing cellular oxygen. It also shrinks tumors and increases the effects of other drugs. Curcumin and ECGC work together synergistically and make each other stronger.

Step 3
K2 as Mk-4
Note: Do not take if you are on blood thinners
Why: Because it works on a cellular level, it can burn up and process the cancer toxins, growth and kill the cells without making the body process any carcinogens directly through bowel movements.

Step 4
Milk Thistle (Silymarin)
Why: Because it works to assist curcumin without interfering with how curcumin interrupts and kills cancer but also kills cancer itself. It helps with liver detoxification which allows the body to

better eliminate ammonia from the cancer and mycotoxins released. It assists to prevent further DNA damage. It can work as a standalone treatment or in combination but in combination works better. If your body is to weak for Curcumin, Silymarin is a good replacement at the correct dosage.

Step 5
Q10 as Ubiquinol

WARNING: DO NOT USE Q10 IF YOU ARE PLANNING ON CHEMOTHERAPY OR RADIATION.
Why: The First step to any cancer is not what you put in your body, it is your body itself. Everyone has carcinogens in their body, the trick is how your body removes them. If the Cells inside your body have dysfunctional DNA, your body cannot remove the bad cells and if the cells have no control over replication which is the second step, then you will indeed get cancer. What controls all this process in the cells you got it "Coenzyme q10". It is not a standalone but it is the start of the journey and the root of the problem. Coenzyme 10 is reduced by age, toxins, medicines, chemotherapy and the list goes on.

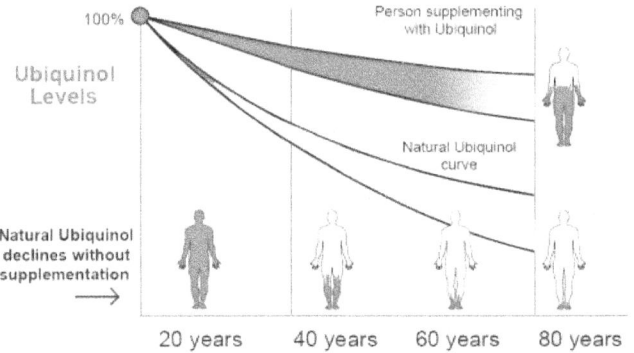

Coq10 induces cell energy, oxygen and metabolism of the cell. It causes tumor remission (apoptosis - self-destruction - of the cancer cell).It reverses cell damage and allows the body to stimulate the immune system and program the cancer cells themselves to kill each other which is very important because it is the part of the cell DNA that causes multiplication of cancer cells. Coq10 inhibits oxidation due to its powerful antioxidant abilities.

DISCLAIMER

www.ingramcontent.com/pod-product-compliance
Lightning Source LLC
Chambersburg PA
CBHW070759180526
45168CB00004B/1679